70 TIPS TO BURN THE FAT

By

FUNMILOLA ADEBOLA

Copyright © 2022 Funmilola Adebola

All rights reserved.

ISBN: 9798846093218

DEDICATION

This book is dedicated to my family. My supportive husband, whose words of inspiration and prodding for tenacity echo in my ear, deserves a personal expression of gratitude. I will always be grateful for everything they did. I especially dedicate his book to my spouse for helping me advance my technological knowledge in preparation for the several hours I spent editing.

Table of Contents

ACKNOWLEDGMENTS

I can't thank the Almighty God enough for his unwavering encouragement and support. I want to express my gratitude for the teaching opportunities he has given me.

Additionally, I couldn't have finished this book without the help of my kids, Henry and Kim. I appreciate you letting me spend some time away from you researching and writing. You should all take a trip to Sweden! Thank you also to Mr. and Mrs. Adebola, who are my parents. We won't soon forget the numerous occasions you looked after the kids while we had busy schedules.

Finally, I want to express my sincere appreciation to Prince Olajide, my loving, supportive, and caring husband. Your words of support during trying times were greatly appreciated and duly remembered. Knowing that you were willing to manage our household tasks while I finished my work was a wonderful comfort and relief. My sincere appreciation!

INTRODUCTION

There was a time in our society when eating what mom made for dinner and going to work the only options. The difference between that culture and ours is that people in the former worked on their feet in the fields or on a warehouse floor, not in front of a computer screen. The only way to work, and the reason it was termed work, was through physical labor. People could frequently eat everything they wanted during this time since they were burning off significantly more calories than they were taking in.

But like all good things, which has come to an end, and thanks to modern technology, we are now all overweight. Our comfort levels have grown tenfold, and our lives have changed so radically. Every rose has its thorn, as they say, and in our society, our desire for luxurious lifestyles and less work has started to show around the waistline.

The unfortunate aspect of it all is that the danger increases as your weight increases. If you don't do anything about it, illness—whether it takes the shape of diabetes or a heart condition—is guaranteed to manifest. Prior to reaching the point when you can no longer control your weight, you must be proactive in losing weight. It's not necessarily important to have a toned and sculpted body, but rather to be at a healthy weight. The abs

can be worked on later; for now, you only need to lose a little additional body fat. People are attempting to lose weight as society becomes aware of what is happening and that we are all overweight. The abs can be worked on later; for now, you only need to lose a little more body fat. People are attempting to play catch up and operate from a position of weakness as society becomes aware of what is occurring and that we are overweight as a culture. They want to live a healthy lifestyle and shed some pounds.

You can focus on your abs later; for now, all you need to do is lose a little extra body fat. People are attempting to play catch up and work from behind as society becomes aware of what is happening and that we are all overweight. They want to have a better lifestyle and lose weight.

People fail to recognize that the first step in shedding the initial 10 pounds is what they consume. In reality, most people are unaware that they may mistakenly believe they are hungry when they are truly dehydrated and actually thirsty. Water is also marvelous. Water alone makes up more than 66 percent of your body weight. Water is essential for maintaining a healthy weight for the same reason.

Chapter 1

Exercising to Lose weight

TIP 1

Play some basketball or tennis. A wonderful approach to get in shape is to play video games. Working out with a friend in a competitive setting is also more enjoyable. If you push yourself harder, you'll burn more calories; just be careful not to overdo it.

TIP 2

When you can, go swimming. For those with osteoporosis or joint issues, swimming is a terrific aerobic workout because it has little to no impact on your joints.

TIP 3

Join a dancing class. This can involve learning ballroom dances like the fox trot, salsa, or tango. These fast-moving dances will have you moving. Ballroom dancing is vigorous workout and will tone your legs even when done slowly. Alternately, enroll

in an aerobic dancing class. How many overweight dancers are you familiar with?

TIP 4

Give your partner a massage. If they have been working out with you, you can exert a small bit of yourself while also praising them for the weight they have shed.

TIP 5

Instead of going up the stairs one at a time, go up them twice. Your heart rate goes up as a result of having to push yourself more.

TIP 6

Take a walk with your dog. If you're not exercising enough, there's a good chance your pet isn't either. Alternately, let your dog walk you. Allow him to lead you for once in his life in the direction and at the pace he chooses. It may be beneficial.

TIP 7

Push your body away from the wall with your hands while leaning against it with your face near to it. S

TIP 8

Give yoga a try. Yoga is a fantastic method to get in shape and relieve tension. Through yoga, you can learn to manage your muscles and increase the control you have over each specific muscle group.

TIP 9

People underestimate the amount of fat that strength training can burn. When you work on developing muscle, your body starts to burn fat as fuel for your growing muscles. Be aware that because muscle weighs more than fat, your scale might not accurately reflect your weight loss as you add muscle.

TIP 10

Suck in your stomach when you walk. Walk properly, but do your best to keep that stomach tucked in. You will soon begin to feel those muscles tightening.

TIP 11

Do breathing exercises to tone your midsection. It is amazing how breathing properly and with your entire diaphragm can actually help to tighten your abdominal muscles. Most people breathe way too shallow as it is and oxygen is good for the brain.

TIP 12

Avoid drinking excessive amounts of coffee, as it desensitizes your body to the natural fat burning effects that caffeine has. One or two cups (if the day's really slow to get started) max.

TIP 13

Play some music and get up and move. It goes without saying that the more you move, the better you'll feel and the more weight you'll shed.

TIP 14

If you're on the bus or train, get off a few blocks before your stop and continue walking from there. This is a convenient method to get in a walk before and after work or en route to somewhere else.

TIP 15

To tone your midsection, use pelvic gyrations. These are obviously not exercises you would perform in public, but they are a fantastic first step in getting your body ready for more challenging stomach crunches. It keeps you lose rather than tight and is also helpful for your back muscles.

TIP 16

Keep the remote out of sight. Additionally harmful to weight loss are remote controllers. Without a remote, you might not even turn on the TV, which means you might look for more engaging activities to do. If you don't have a remote, get up and change the station, or go for a walk in place of watching TV.

TIP 17

Do your own fetching. If you need something from the kitchen, the TV channel changed, the mail or newspaper from the driveway, walk and get it yourself. Adding a little walking to your day will do wonders for you.

TIP 18

Walk along or climb the escalator with it or just take the stairs

TIP 19

Move around or perform easy workouts like crunches or leaning over and touching your toes during commercial breaks. Do whatever it takes to keep your blood circulating and your body moving.

TIP 20

While running is one way to obtain your daily 10 minutes of cardio, there are other ways as well.

TIP 21

Try 15 minutes of brisk walking to stay in shape if you are unable to run due to a physical condition.

TIP 21

If you have the time, you can walk almost anyplace. Consider walking or riding a bike if going to work or the store is close by. It may take you longer, but you're getting your workout in at the same time.

Chapter 2

Suggested Weight Loss Plan

TIP 22

Stay away from the couch and the TV to lose weight. Don't sit on it if you have a tendency to turn into a couch potato. To avoid wasting too much time in front of the television, if necessary, place a less comfortable chair there. If you're a computer addict, the same applies to that device. Some people find that sitting in front of their computer is more comfortable than sitting in front of the television. (Obviously, this only applies to those who are required to spend prolonged periods of time sitting in front of a computer when they do not work from home.

TIP 23

Stand up and stretch every 30 minutes or so if you work a job that requires you to sit for the entire shift. The majority of today's occupations demand you to sit down in front of a computer. Make it a point to move occasionally if you have a job like this.

TIP 24

Pick a workout plan that works for your lifestyle. Everyone has a distinct lifestyle and works in a

different field. There is no specific time that you must or must not exercise. If you find that working out late before bed is calming for you, then do it. It's also fantastic if you prefer to exercise first thing in the morning because it helps you wake up. Due to the stress of their jobs or because it is the only time they have available, some people like working out during their lunch break.

If you can stand, avoid sitting. You can burn more calories by standing than by sitting if you can do it comfortably.

TIP 25

When your body tells you it has had enough, take a break. When you have worked out for a considerable amount of time, you will start receiving signals from your body. This is particularly important when you are just getting started in your exercise routine.

TIP 26

If you decide to increase the length of your workouts, do so gradually. The same is true for the intensity of your workouts.

TIP 27

Collect information on exercise and easy things you can do from your own home. There is tons of extensive research available on exercise and you can choose what will assist you the most to meet your weight loss goals. Browse the Internet or pick up some books on health and exercise from your local bookstore or library to learn more and how to burn

off the desired number of calories you are trying to burn each week.

TIP 28

Try to find an exercise buddy. This should be someone who is as committed to exercising and losing weight as you are. One of the advantages of finding a committed partner is that you have someone to keep feeling responsible to them. The knowledge that someone is waiting on you makes it easier for you to get out of bed and go exercise with them. You wouldn't want to stand up your exercise buddy would you?

TIP 29

You can maintain your weight with three days of 30 minutes of exercise, but to start losing weight, you need at least four days of 30 minutes of activity, and five days a week is even better.

TIP 30

Gather knowledge on exercises and simple tasks you may complete at home. There is a ton of in-depth research on exercise accessible, and you may chose what will help you the most to achieve your weight loss objectives. For further information on how to burn the target number of calories you want to burn each week, browse the web or have a look at some books on health and fitness that are available at your local library or bookstore.

TIP 31

Reward yourself when you frequently check your

weight and the way your clothes fit. Purchase a new pair of pants or a new pair of running shoes for yourself. As you work toward your weight loss objectives, this will support you in staying motivated. Take a day off from working out to give your body a chance to recover and mend. Every week, your body requires a day off.

When you begin exercising, weigh yourself, but don't take the results as a gauge for how much weight you are losing. Your weight changes over the course of the day. If you weigh yourself every day, you might simply end up giving up.

TIP 32

Don't give up if you don't notice results immediately away when you start working out, whether at home or in a gym. To start improving and getting your body into shape, it takes longer than a week. Many people make the error of thinking that their exercise is ineffective when it only requires a brief period of time.

When you initially start exercising, injuries may result from pushing your body too far. Your ligaments, joints, and bones are not designed to withstand the strain you are placing on them. Do not believe that if you really push yourself during a few workouts that you will lose money; sadly, this is not how the body functions. Slow and steady wins the race.

Chapter 3

Change Your Cooking Style to Lose Weight

There are two things you must do in order to lose weight, and one of them—eating healthy foods and drinking enough of pure water—has already been described in great detail here. Get your body moving as the other thing you need to accomplish .Exercise doesn't require you to buy a gym membership. In truth, there are a number of daily activities you may engage in to help your body start losing weight, as well as a number of workouts you can perform alone to accomplish so.

TIP 33

Whether it's liquid meals, desserts, or ice cream, chew it at least 8 to 12 times. Saliva is added to the food, aiding in the sugar's digestion. When food isn't thoroughly chewed and is instead just swallowed, you flood your stomach with indigestible food that doesn't provide the necessary health advantages.

TIP 34

Use high-quality extra virgin olive oil while cooking using oil, according to Tip #51. It is more expensive than vegetable oil, but because of the superior health advantages, the price is justified. Olive oil helps to strengthen the suppleness of the arterial walls, which lowers the possibility of developing coronary heart disease and has been linked to a reduced risk of it.

TIP 35

Avoid foods with no or low fat content. These food products are widely available, although they are not particularly healthful. Many of these foods are sweetened with a chemical or carbohydrate to improve their flavor. These substances and carbohydrates are nevertheless converted by the body into sugar, which implies that fat is still formed from them.

TIP 36

Avoid being a victim of crash diets. These are detrimental to your health and ultimately cause more harm than good. Usually, you will drop a few pounds in the short term, but as soon as you stop, everything returns, making your weight worse than before.

TIP 37

Instead of frying in oil or fat, try baking those items instead. Baking does not require all the fat and oil that frying requires and your food is not soaking in those substances while it cooks.

TIP 38

Use non-stick frying pan spray so you don't use oil. Also, pans that are non-stick don't require as much, if any oil.

TIP 39

Boil vegetables instead of cooking them. You can also steam them, as this is probably the healthiest way to eat foods like cabbages, cauliflower, broccoli and carrots.

TIP 40

Use less salt overall and make an effort to reduce it in half. One of the biggest contributors to obesity is salt.

TIP 41

Try grazing five to six times each day .These are the snacks that we previously spoke about. Some people find that they lose weight more successfully when they never feel hungry, and you can achieve this by grazing on healthy foods. Additionally, it keeps your metabolism active, which naturally burns fat.

TIP 42

Don't worry about cheating, but avoid doing so during meals. Consume treats and your favorite cheat food solely for flavor. Share a dessert with the entire family if you desire one after dinner. You won't gain any weight, just the flavor.

TIP 43

Watch your fat intake. A gram of fat contains 9 calories. You can calculate the quantity of fat in those things if you know your overall calorie intake.

TIP 44

Multigrain breads with high fiber content are significantly preferable to white bread. These breads provide a significant amount of protein and are another option to increase the fiber in your diet.

TIP 45

Eating pork in no way helps you lose weight. When attempting to lose weight, it is best to consume less pork. Foods like bacon, ham, and sausage are made from pork, which also has a high fat content.

TIP 46

Try to cut back as much as you can on sugar. Try to discover an artificial sweetener whose flavor you don't mind if you must add sweetness to your coffee and tea. These activities, however, should be avoided because they are not very healthful.

TIP 47

Between 15 and 20 percent of your meal should include fats. This is all the fat your body actually need. You'll be eating a lot of this in the diet in the form of cream, sugar, and other things.

TIP 48

Eat more white meat than red meat. Chicken, fish, and some other poultry are examples of white flesh. Beef and pork are examples of red meat.

TIP 49

Try to eat as many vegetarian meals as you can. Even if you can't entirely cut out meat, this is still a better way of living. The better is to consume as many fruits and vegetables as you can. The more meat you eliminate from your diet, the fatter you may eliminate as well. However, protein is crucial, so be sure your choice

TIP 50

Try to have breakfast an hour after waking up . The greatest method to give your body the boost it needs is to do this. Avoid waiting till you are genuinely hungry. Although breakfast is crucial, you shouldn't overeat. You're supposed to be breaking your fast after not eating all night.

TIP 51

All food groups, including carbohydrates, should be present in your diet. In actuality, 50–55 percent of your diet must consist of carbohydrates. A significant source of energy is carbs. Diets that forbid carbs are harmful to you and just increase your cravings for them. You shouldn't lack any nutrients due to your diet.

TIP 52

Only 25 to 30 percent of your diet should consist of proteins.

TIP 53

Limit your egg consumption to one per day. The best option is to limit your egg consumption to three per week.

TIP 54

Treat chocolates like a luxury good. Purchase the best, and consume them infrequently. Each bite will taste even better if you actually take the time to appreciate it. This will increase your enjoyment of the meal.

TIP 55

Include foods from each food group in your daily diet. This is a fantastic technique to make sure you are getting all the nutrients your body need and it aids in preventing any dietary deficits. Additionally, avoid eating the same things repeatedly. Try new things to avoid getting bored with your current diet.

Don't skip meals—tip number 27. A minimum of three meals each day are recommended, but five small meals are preferred. As a result, you won't become ravenous during the day and end up overeating.

TIP 56

Fresh vegetables are preferable to canned ones, just like fruits. If you can eat your vegetables raw, that is

even better. The nutrients are lost when you cook them. If you must cook them, try to boil them just long enough to keep some of their crispness. Don't dunk them in butter either. It would be best if you could purchase organic vegetables free of pesticides.

TIP 57

For those foods that are a need, counting calories is a good idea. If the food is packed, the calories will be listed on the packaging. Make careful to consider the caloric content of serving sizes as well. Because an Otis Spunk Meyer muffin is meant to be two servings, you must multiply the calorie count by two. Here is where food producers start to play shady, and you must not fall for their tricks.

TIP 58

Work off the additional calories by the end of the week. Make sure to visit the gym or go for a longer walk if you feel like you have indulged excessively this week in order to burn off those additional calories.

TIP 59

Only eat if you are truly hungry. Make careful to first sip on some water to ascertain whether you are truly thirsty or truly hungry. It's common for people to eat when they see food. They simply want to consume it; it does not imply that they are hungry. If you're not truly hungry, don't accept any food that is offered to you. If you feel obligated to eat it out of politeness, simply nibble; skip a meal.

TIP 60

Try to avoid snacking in between meals, but if you must, make sure it's a healthy snack. Try to find healthy snacks rather than junk food if you travel frequently.

TIP 61

Control your sweet tooth. You can still enjoy your favorite sweets as long as you don't consume them as a meal. Always keep in mind that these treats contribute to a situation that you don't want them to contribute to. However, don't deprive yourself either because you'll eat twice as much as you ought to.

TIP 62

Set a time for meals and stick to it. Try to schedule your meals so that you can consume them at those times. You can manage when and what you eat by developing an eating routine. Additionally, eating five little meals throughout the day is preferable to just one or two large ones. One meal a day is all your body needs.

TIP 63

Make informed food choices. Eat just when you are hungry. Animals eat out of instinct, but humans only eat when they are aware that their bodies are truly hungry. Avoid impulsive eating.

TIP 64

Be mindful of everything you eat, from the dish

itself to the garnishes. A healthy dinner might be ruined by garnishes and condiments because they frequently include a lot of fat.

TIP 65

Veggies are your friends if you're trying to lose weight. There are many options available here, and you might even wish to try ones that you haven't tried before. The greatest types of greens are leafy, and you should always incorporate salads into your meals when you can. As long as you don't drown them in cheese and excessive dressing, salads are nutrient-rich meals. There is a lot of natural water in the leafy greens as well.

TIP 66

Consume water-rich fresh produce like fruits and vegetables. These include items such as tomatoes, watermelons, cantaloupe, kiwi, grapes, etc. All of those luscious, fresh fruits and vegetables are healthy for you. You may consume a lot of these foods without gaining weight because they are between 90 and 95 percent water.

TIP 67

Choose fresh fruit over fruit that has been processed. Anything that is converted into additional sugar. Processed and canned fruits also do not have as much fiber as fresh fruits.

TIP 68

Increase your fiber intake as much as you can. This usually means eating more fruits and veggies.

Eating healthfully and shedding pounds

Okay, so the majority of people think of diets when they consider reducing weight and eating. Unfortunately, weight gain is a common side effect of all popular diets. Why? Because after being starved to death, the victim finally succumbs to their hunger and consumes everything in sight. They also deny them their favorite foods. This is not a healthy way to eat or a way to live. You only put yourself under stress, which makes you eat more.

So, there are a few guidelines for eating well that you may use every day without having to give up the things you enjoy.

TIP 69

Don't drink too much tea or coffee. If you don't add a lot of cream and sugar to them, they are essentially safe. The cream and sugar turn into fatty ingredients. Consider it this way: Every time you drink a cup of coffee or tea with cream and two sugar cubes, it's like eating a piece of chocolate cake. Imagine how much cake you will consume after drinking a Venti Starbucks Latte; ouch.

TIP 70

Try to avoid soda as much as possible. All sodas are heavily sugar sweetened. It's best to eliminate as much of your diet as you can. Diet soda is still soda, too. Despite having less sugar, it still contains additional chemicals and ingredients that are bad for your health. When consuming soda, follow it up with a glass of water. Keep in mind that caffeine also

dehydrates you. Sodas that have been decaffeinated still include small levels of caffeine and the same amount of sugar, making them not significantly healthier.

Chapter 4

Get Cracking

Now that you know how to get started, read on for some further advice on how to lose weight and keep it off, which all starts with what you eat.

Due to the fact that we are currently at an all-time high in our level of obesity, weight reduction and fat are such crucial aspects of our lives. Anybody listening in on a discussion or watching television will pay attention when the word "weight loss programs" is spoken. That's actually one of the most frequently searched keywords on the web right now.

Our relationship with food is the fundamental explanation of why we are so overweight. In our culture, we frequently place an emphasis on quantity. Instead of the best cuisine available, we simply want as much as we can obtain. When it should be the exact opposite, quantity always triumphs over quality.

It might be challenging to decide where to start once you've made the decision to reduce weight. It is achievable if you have a strong desire to start working out and lose weight. You simply need to learn how to refuse requests.

Everyone is unique. Nobody one will have the same metabolism as you or burn fat in the same manner as you do. Even if you started an exercise and diet

regimen at the same time as the person next to you and followed the same routine every day, you could not see the same results two weeks or even a month later. Having said that, it's crucial to understand that not everyone uses food in the same manner. What might make one individual gain a pound might not make another do the same.

The same is true when trying to lose weight. Even if you eat and exercise exactly the same, you and your spouse could not have the same outcomes if you're married and working out together. For example, if he stops drinking soda and loses five pounds as a result, but you don't, it proves that you and your husband might not.

The fact is that modern society has a lot more work to do than cultures in the past. Women and men were skinny sixty years ago because they had to work. You had to perform manual labor if you wanted to eat. If you wanted eggs, you had to go fetch them from the hen coop. If you wanted fresh milk, you had to go milk the cows. And if you wanted to cultivate vegetables, you had to plow the fields. You had to be aware of the process of rearing a calf and having it killed if you desired beef. That was the way things were back then, but all of this laborious labor has been eliminated by technology.

As a result, we must monitor our diet and force ourselves to exercise. If we don't, half the time we have no cause to move.

It is crucial to realize how much work you are willing to put into achieving your weight loss

objectives. It is the only goal in life that requires physical exertion if you want to see results.

Typically, people do not have to worry about weight loss until they are in their twenties, but with the prevalence of fast food in our culture today, this is not always the case. Because they eat too much fast food and processed food, many of our kids are obese. Read the components of the food you are consuming when you go grocery shopping for yourself and your family. Don't consume anything you can't say out loud. We acquire weight as a result of our cravings, which are triggered by processed foods. If you want to successfully lose weight and keep it off in the future, you must fully comprehend this.

However, merely monitoring your diet won't result in weight loss. The right diet must be combined with the right volume of exercise. The answer is to follow an exercise routine that will provide your body with the workout it needs to burn calories and fat effectively. If you don't move around, it's as though you're in hibernation and your body just continues to put on weight, especially around your waist.

Chapter 5

Exercise is Beneficial to You.

It just makes you feel nice all over when you recall a time when the sun and hard work were the causes of your sweat. You feel stronger all over as a result of the sun's direct impact on your shoulders and the tension it places on your muscles. Working out outside is the best thing.

The majority of people no longer work on farms, but a small number still get to experience the joy of doing work, creating something tangible, and maintaining a healthy weight while doing it. How many farm workers, cowboys, and ranchers are overweight, really? It really is a healthy way of living. Unfortunately, the majority of us spend our days sitting down inside working while continuing to consume three meals per day, often without the chance to really enjoy them.

Except for those who live in cities where they can walk everywhere, it is a fact of life that city dwellers don't get much exercise. This implies that you must work hard and set your mind to it. You must incorporate exercise into your everyday routine to

avoid being overweight and ill. It simply so happens that way. Exercise is the best approach to treat obesity, stress, hypertension, cardio vascular disease, and other disorders linked to a sedentary lifestyle.

Chapter 6

Equilibrium Key

The most crucial component of any fitness program is consistency. You can achieve your goals if you set them and continually work toward them.

Most people find it simple to start. They go shopping, purchase some active wear, running shoes, and perhaps a gym membership. After that, they engage in fairly consistent exercise for a week or two.

Even though many people prefer to exercise in the evenings, other people find it more difficult to stick with this schedule. This is an excellent time to leave if you are not entirely worn out when you get off work. However, if you are unable to, you might need to figure out a way to travel there in the morning. You'll be able to stay consistent and it will assist you get awake.

www.ingramcontent.com/pod-product-compliance
Lightning Source LLC
LaVergne TN
LVHW020536160826
845677LV00015B/4096

* 9 7 9 8 8 4 6 0 9 3 2 1 8 *